Supplement 3 zu Band 23, April 2000

Offizielles Organ der Deutschen Gesellschaft für Hämatologie und Onkologie, der Österreichischen Gesellschaft für Hämatologie und Onkologie, der Österreichischen Krebsgesellschaft – Krebsliga unter Fortführung der «Österreichischen Zeitung für Onkologie»

ONKOLOGIE

• International Journal for Cancer Research and Treatment

KARGER

Basel · Freiburg · Paris · London · New York · New Delhi · Bangkok · Singapore · Tokyo · Sydney

Bibliographische Dienste
Biological Abstracts
Current Contents/Clinical Medicine
Excerpta Medica/EMBASE
Medical Documentation Service
Reference Update
Research Alert
Science Citation Index
SCISEARCH Database

S. Karger · Medical and Scientific Publishers · Basel · Freiburg · Paris · London · New York · New Delhi · Bangkok · Singapore · Tokyo · Sydney

Die Zeitschrift erscheint zweimonatlich; pro Jahr erscheint 1 Band zu je 6 Heften. Bezugspreis für Jahrgang 23, 2000, DEM 218,– / CHF 170,–, einschließlich MwSt., zuzüglich Postgebühren. Der Abonnementpreis ist im voraus zahlbar. Das Abonnement der Zeitschrift läuft weiter, wenn es nicht spätestens 4 Wochen vor Abschluß eines Bandes abbestellt wird.
Abonnementbestellungen können bei jeder Buchhandlung oder direkt beim Verlag aufgegeben werden:
Deutschland: S. Karger GmbH, Lörracher Str. 16a, D-79115 Freiburg, Telefon +49 7 61 45 20 70, Telefax +49 7 61 4 52 07 14, E-mail Information@Karger.de, Postbank München 400 80-807.
Übrige Länder: S. Karger AG, Allschwilerstr. 10, Postfach, CH-4009 Basel, Telefon +41 61 3 06 11 11, Telefax +41 61 3 06 12 34, E-mail Karger@Karger.ch.

Anzeigen: S. Karger Verlag für Medizin und Naturwissenschaften GmbH, Lörracher Str. 16a, D-79115 Freiburg, Telefon +49 7 61 45 20 70.
Gültig ist die Preisliste Nr. 10 vom 1. Januar 1999.
Für den Inhalt außerhalb des redaktionellen Teiles (insbesondere Anzeigen, Industrieinformationen, Pressezitate und Kongreßinformationen) übernehmen Schriftleitung, Beirat und Verlag keine Gewähr.

Supplement 3 zu Band 23, April 2000; ISBN 3-8055-7088-0

Verlagsleitung und presserechtlich verantwortlich: Sibylle Hopf
Anzeigenleitung: Susanne Meister
Produktionsleitung: Georg Brunner

Herstellung: Konkordia Druck GmbH, Eisenbahnstraße 31, D-77815 Bühl

KARGER

Fax +49 761 4 52 07 14
E-mail Information@Karger.de
www.karger.com

Home Page der Zeitschrift:
www.karger.com/journals/onk

ONKOLOGIE

Supplement 3 zu Band 23, April 2000

Survival as a Response Criterion for Small-Cell Lung Cancer

Guest-Editors:
P. Drings, Heidelberg, *R. Stahel,* Zürich

KARGER

Basel · Freiburg · Paris · London · New York ·
New Delhi · Bangkok · Singapore · Tokyo · Sydney

Contents · Inhalt

ONKOLOGIE

Vol. 23, Suppl 3, April 2000

KARGER

Fax +49 761 4 52 07 14
E-mail Information@Karger.de
www.karger.com

Artikel (Volltext) und Inhaltsverzeichnisse
sowie das vorläufige Inhaltsverzeichnis des nächsten Heftes:
www.karger.com/journals/onk/onk_bk.htm

Editorial

ONKOLOGIE

Onkologie 2000;23(suppl 3):1

Status of Topotecan in Small-Cell Lung Cancer

P. Drings[a] R. Stahel[b]

[a]Thoraxklinik Heidelberg gGmbH, [b]Labor für Onkologie, Departement Innere Medizin, Universitätsspital Zürich

The presentations of the symposium 'Revisiting Response in SCLC: Advantage with Topotecan?' (Zürich, April 16.–18., 1999) confirm that topotecan belongs to the most potent substances for this tumor entity. The cytostatic drug has been intensively investigated during the last view years. Remission rates in previously untreated patients with extensive disease reach 40% and the median survival time is 10 month. Also in pretreated patients the drug proved its efficacy. In cases with remissions after primary therapy, the remission rate in second-line treatment was 38%, whereas it was only 6.4% in primarily refractory patients.

In the randomized comparison within a phase III study, topotecan proved to be equipotent in the treatment of relapsed patients as a monotherapy compared with the combination of cyclophosphamide, doxorubicin and vincristine (CAV) with respect to remission rates and survival time, and it was even slightly superior with respect to symptom control.

In the meantime, as a logical consequence of its efficiency in the second-line treatment, topotecan has also been used as first-line therapy of small-cell lung cancer. Several studies in the USA and in Germany document the high activity of topotecan in combination with paclitaxel, etoposide or cisplatinum. These studies are currently underway and await final conclusions.

Also interesting is the observation that brain metastases are diminished with this therapy. Possibly, topotecan may develop a protective effect against the clinical manifestation of brain metastasis. In conclusion, topotecan belongs to the most important and inevitable drugs in the treatment of small-cell lung cancer. Up to date, however, its position is only settled beyond any doubt in the second-line treatment. Treatment of the relapse in these patients is frequently difficult and problematic. In this situation, drugs with a good efficacy profile and low side effects are of special advantage.

KARGER

Fax +49 761 4 52 07 14
E-mail Information@Karger.de
www.karger.com

Accessible online at:
www.karger.com/journals/onk

Prof. Dr. P. Drings
Thoraxklinik Heidelberg gGmbH
Amalienstraße 5
D-69126 Heidelberg (Germany)

ONKOLOGIE

Onkologie 2000;23(suppl 3):2–6

Phase I and II Evaluation of Novel Anticancer Agents: Are Response and Toxicity the Right Endpoints?

E. A. Eisenhauer

Investigational New Drug Program, NCIC Clinical Trials Group, Queen's University, Kingston

Introduction

Research into the molecular basis of malignancy has yielded numerous investigational agents directed towards intracellular and extracellular targets. At the level of the cell, agents targeting cytoplasmic and cell surface signaling molecules, processes of cell cycle control, and mutations or lack of expression of suppressor genes are entering the clinic. At the extracellular level, there are large numbers of novel drugs designed to limit tumor penetration and metastasis and agents that directly inhibit angiogenesis. Since many of these compounds may be *cytostatic* rather than *cytotoxic* in their effects on tumor, they present challenges for phase I and II evaluation where traditional endpoints may not be appropriate.

Thus a challenge facing those involved in clinical drug development is the need to reevaluate the conceptual framework we have used for cancer treatment. Although the ultimate goal of cancer therapy, to prolong survival or cure this disease, will not change, our understanding of the mechanism of action of some of these new agents will cause us to shift our treatment approach. The familiar paradigm of giving as high a dose as possible in rounds of cyclical therapy may need to be shifted to one of repeated smaller doses adequate to inhibit the target, but not sufficient to produce serious toxic effects. This paradigm shift leads to challenges at the phase I and II level of drug development with respect to how we select dose and how to detect efficacy if it truly exists. Are there substitutes for toxicity as a means of defining dose recommendations? What can replace tumor regression as an assessment of efficacy in the phase II setting? And can any new proposed endpoints be rendered meaningful by their relationship to survival?

Goals of Phase I and II Trials

Despite the fact that novel agents may present challenges in trial design, the *goals* of phase I and II clinical trials of these agents will remain the same: Phase I trials should determine an appropriate dose and schedule for further evaluation, will describe the pharmacologic behavior of the drug and its toxic effects. The goal of phase II trials will be to screen agents for evidence of antitumor activity. The area that has been generating a great deal of discussion is not the goals of these trials but rather *what endpoints are available to assess them*.

Alternative Endpoints for Phase I Trials

In the case of standard cytotoxic agents, the observation of both dose-response and dose-toxicity relationships in preclinical studies led to the use of toxicity as a phase I endpoint and the goal of delivering the highest doses possible. In this context, toxicity has been seen as a surrogate for doses that might be effective. Whether the same approach is rational for newer agents should depend on the preclinical data: A *plateau* on the dose-efficacy curve or a *dissociation* between doses that are effective and those which are toxic implies toxic doses may be neither necessary nor desirable (see fig. 1 for examples). If

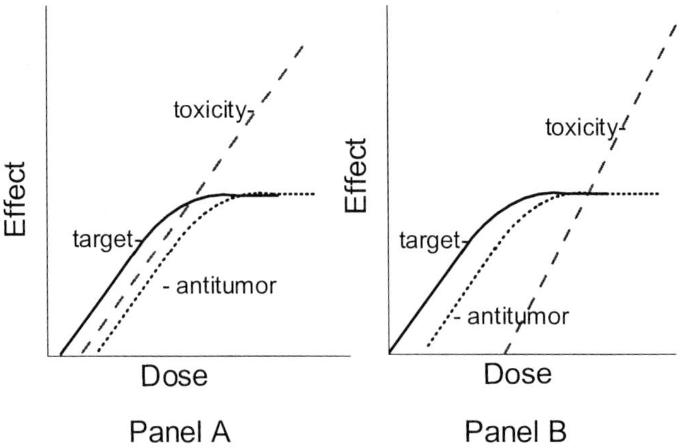

Fig. 1. Preclinical data (idealized) which may exist for some novel agents. See text for explanation of panels A and B.

KARGER

Fax +49 761 4 52 07 14
E-mail Information@Karger.de
www.karger.com

Accessible online at:
www.karger.com/journals/onk

Dr. Elizabeth Eisenhauer
Director, Investigational New Drug Program
NCIC Clinical Trials Group, Queen's University
Kingston, Ontario Canada K7L 3N6
Fax 1-613-533-2411
E-mail: eeisenhauer@ctg.queensu.ca

Table 1. Potential alternative phase I endpoints

Measures of target effect
In tumor
In normal tissue
Direct
Indirect
Surrogates for activity
Especially vaccine studies
Blood levels
Toxicity

Target Effect	Significant Toxicity	
	Seen	Not Seen
Inhibition	Continue	Continue
No Inhibition	Continue or stop?	Stop

Fig. 2. Possible outcomes of phase I trials with new endpoints. How to integrate findings of toxicity and target effects in decisions regarding continued development?

Table 2. Phase I trials of novel agents: My view

1. Measure toxicity, blood levels and if available, target effect
2. Design trial with two MTDs:
   a. Maximum target inhibiting dose (MTID)
   b. Maximum tolerated dose (MTD)
3. If same: select dose for further evaluation
4. If different: choose dose with less toxicity, but maximum target effect. Consider comparison!

toxic effects are mediated by a different mechanism than the targeted antitumor effect, increasing doses to toxic levels may not be necessary to achieve efficacy.

There are several endpoints that may be alternatives to toxicity for agents showing these relationships. These include measurement of target inhibition, measurements of surrogates for activity, and assessment of drug levels in plasma (table 1). Toxicity is still relevant of course because it may limit dosing on its own, so it cannot be omitted.

Measurement of effect on the molecular target is particularly appealing because of its rational basis, but the challenges to its use as an endpoint for phase I evaluation are many. How and in which tissues to measure 'target effect' should be based on preclinical data validating the proposed clinical measurement, i.e. the effect on target in the tissue to be sampled should correlate with efficacy. The relevant tissue in which to measure target inhibition is tumor and this is seldom available in repeated patient samples. Available tissue, which is usually blood or other normal tissue such as buccal mucosa, may not be relevant. At the very least, if normal cells are to be used to evaluate the magnitude of target inhibition, there ought to be evidence from preclinical models that target inhibition in that tissue type is a valid marker for efficacy. This is often not the case. Furthermore, species specificity of molecular inhibitors may make this type of assessment impossible. How one measures the effect on the target is also a subject for debate. Should the target inhibition be measured directly (e.g.: decreased production of a specific targeted protein) or indirectly (e.g.: measurement of proteins or products downstream from the target itself?) Either approach requires intensive laboratory back up, and if the measure selected is to be a phase I endpoint, these assays must be done in 'real-time' fashion to allow decisions about subsequent dose escalation. A weakness of this approach may relate to the target itself. Although preclinical data may suggest that an agent's efficacy is due to interaction with a specific target, it is certainly plausible that it may have other, as yet unknown, effects at the cellular level responsible for its antitumor activity. Thus the target that we believe is relevant (and strive to measure) may not be responsible for antitumor effect.

Measurement of surrogates for activity is another possible endpoint for phase I evaluation. This is of particular interest for immune-based treatments where measures of immune response may be dose-dependent and predict for efficacy. The major challenge in this context is to define *which* measures are truly related to antitumor effect. Preclinical models may help, but immune therapies are often species-specific, limiting the assessment of appropriate surrogates in the lab. Furthermore, multiple measurements of immune function may generate discordant results leading to confusion in interpretation.

Measurement of blood levels of drug and toxic effects are simpler phase I endpoints. Although as noted earlier, administering toxic doses may not be *necessary*, it is almost certainly the case that a dose high enough to produce toxic effects will not be too *low* for efficacy. Furthermore it is reasonable to suppose that blood levels correlating with target inhibition and with efficacy in animal models could be extrapolated to the clinical situation. Even if measures of target inhibition are possible, toxicity and pharmacologic data must still be collected.

If some measure of target inhibition as well as usual blood level and toxicity information can be obtained, how will these results be integrated into decisions about the future development of a new agent? Figure 2 illustrates the various outcome scenarios possible following completion of phase I trials. In the presence of dose-limiting toxicity together with evidence of target inhibition, further drug development ought to proceed. The same decision would also be rational if dose-related target inhibition were achieved without severe toxicity. The observation of neither toxic effects *nor* evidence of inhibition should lead to concern about the continued evaluation of the compound. The most difficult of all scenarios, I believe, is when dose-limiting toxicity is seen but no inhibition at the tar-

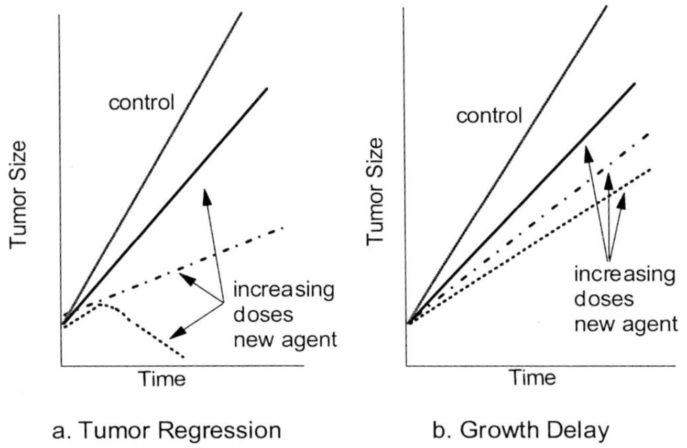

Fig. 3. Patterns of antitumor effects seen in preclinical experiments. Growth delay may be more commonly seen with novel agents than with traditional cytotoxics.

get level has been noted. Here, a decision about whether to move forward into phase II will depend on the certainty with which the true target is known and the strength of the preclinical efficacy data.

Table 2 illustrates my views on the design of phase I trials with non-cytotoxic agents. If possible toxicity, blood levels and target effect should all be measured. Ideally the trial could be designed with two MTDs: the maximum target inhibiting dose (MTID) and the more traditional maximum tolerated dose (MTD). If at the end of the study, the MTID and MTD are similar, selection of the dose for further evaluation is simple. If they are substantially different, it may be most appropriate to select the dose with lower toxicity but maximum target effect for further evaluation. Consideration should be given, however, to comparing these two doses early on for efficacy in a randomized (phase II) study. Only in this way will we discover which strategic approach (MTID or MTD) is correct.

Alternative Endpoints for Phase II Trials

After completion of phase I trials, the major goal of subsequent clinical evaluation is to define the efficacy of the new compound. Efficacy generally means improvement in survival, cure rates or quality of life. Traditionally, small-sample-size, uncontrolled phase II trials have been utilized to 'screen' agents before designing the large-sample-size randomized trials necessary to definitively establish efficacy. Objective response, arbitrarily defined as at least a 50% decrease in the sum of products of measurable lesions, observed in a minimum number of patients, has been found to be a useful tool in selecting or rejecting agents in phase II. It is important to highlight that response on its own is not 'proof' of efficacy, rather it is useful as a phase II endpoint because it has allowed us to *select drugs or regimens which have subsequently been shown to be effective by prolonging survival.* Although only randomized trials can unequivocally show a survival impact, non-randomized trials remain important as a means of screening agents for their potential in this regard.

Table 3. Potential alternative phase II endpoints

Tumor marker changes:
Fall
Change in rate of rise
Measure of target inhibition
PET scanning changes
Time to progression
Progression rate

If, as shown in figure 3 (left panel), a new agent produces tumor regression in animal models, it is reasonable to expect it will do it in the clinical situation as well. Under these circumstances, response remains the most useful phase II endpoint. The more common scenario is that of growth delay, rather than tumor regression, as shown in the right panel of figure 3. Two general approaches are possible in dealing with this latter profile: 1) identify surrogate endpoints, other than response, which can be used in phase II 'screening' trials or, 2) proceed directly to phase III studies.

Because there are considerable resource, time and ethical advantages to having positive phase II data in hand before moving to phase III, there has been a great deal of interest in identifying valid alternatives to response as phase II endpoints. Possible candidate endpoints include: changes in tumor markers, measures of target inhibition, positron emission tomography (PET) scanning, time to progression, and proportion of patients with early progression (table 3). It is important to note that any proposed alternative endpoint must be viewed as experimental because, until now, only response has been utilized to successfully identify active agents. That is, none of the proposed alternatives have been used alone to select agents later shown to be useful in prolonging survival.

Tumor markers have the advantage of being well described and easily measured. Unfortunately, as noted above, no marker used alone has been validated as a phase II endpoint. Although Rustin et al. [1] suggested that in ovarian cancer, CA-125 might substitute for response rate, these data were generated in studies where the drugs *also* produced tumor regression. It is not known in the case of a cytostatic agent whether a fall in marker will occur without tumor regression *and* whether this allows the selection of survival-enhancing drugs. In addition to exploring fall in marker levels, another research group has suggested that a change in the *rate of rise* in marker may be a useful endpoint for identifying an active agent [2]. In their studies of a metalloproteinase inhibitor, some patients showed a decline in the pre-treatment rate of rise of serum marker; an effect which also seemed to demonstrate a dose-response relationship. Randomized trials with this agent are proceeding and may contribute to the validation of this particular endpoint. A last word of caution: If measurement of markers is proposed as a surrogate for activity, it must be assured that there is not a direct effect of the investigational agent on marker levels through changes in secretion unrelated to tumor burden as was the case with suramin [3]. Measurement of target inhibition is appealing from a scientific point of view but since many novel agents target molecules of, as yet, hypothetical importance in human tumor growth, their inhibition has not yet shown relationship to efficacy in the clinical setting. As noted earlier, these may be more logically an endpoint of phase I trials, where optimizing the dose and schedule is the major goal.

PET scanning is a nuclear medicine technique which uses radiopharmaceuticals such as 2-^{18}flouro-2-deoxy-D-glucose to identify changes in tumor metabolism predictive of subsequent tumor shrinkage [4]. However, if PET scanning can only detect changes when tumor regression (i.e.: response) occurs, then this costly test is not really an alternative to response. Does effective cytostatic therapy produce changes in tumors assessed by PET scanning when response is *not* documented? This is certainly possible, but needs to be explored further.

Although time to progression has the advantage of being a well-described and standardized endpoint in randomized trials, it is difficult to interpret when there is no control group and patient numbers are limited as is the case in a phase II setting.

Progression rate, the proportion of patients who progress in the first 8 weeks of therapy and thus have a 'best response' of progression, is a related idea that has come from work done by the NCIC Clinical Trials Group. We have been interested in exploring progression rate as a possible endpoint for phase II trials.

This idea has come from two different avenues of work. In an evaluation of phase II stopping rules, we have shown that certain drugs could be appropriately declared inactive when one considered not only the number of responses but also the number of progressions in the first cohort of patients in a phase II trial [5, 6 and unpublished data]. That is, even if the critical one response was seen in the first 15 patients, a high number of patients with progression of disease (PD) in the same group indicated the drug was unlikely to have meaningful activity and it would be appropriate to stop the trial early.

Other information of importance in generating this idea came from the observation that, at least in some studies, best responses of partial response and stable disease appear to have a similar impact on survival. A trial in non-small cell lung cancer (NSCLC) which demonstrated that two different regimens of platinum-based chemotherapy, both offered a survival advantage over best supportive care, had relatively low response rates (15 and 25% in the chemotherapy arms) [7]. Thus it was puzzling that the treatment had an impact on overall survival. The analysis of survival by best response category provided the answer: patients with either partial response or stable disease had identical outcomes [8]. Thus the gain in survival was

Table 4. Using PD rate to select new agents

Set maximum PD rate above which agent will be rejected
PD rate of interest will vary according to tumor type as does response rate now
For example:

Tumor type	Response rate of interest, %	PD rate of interest, %
Breast	> 30	< 20
NSCLC	> 20	< 30
Glioma	> 10	< 40

Table 5. Data from NCIC CTG phase II trials

Tumor type	Agent	Observed response rate, %	Observed PD rate, %
Breast (first line)			
	Docetaxel	**55***	**11***
	DPPE/doxorubicin	**50***	**10***
	10-EDAM	**41***	**19***
	Menogaril p.o.	23	23
	Menogaril i.v.	26	43
NSCLC (first line)			
	MTA	**23***	**27***
	Paclitaxel/ifos	15	**27***
	Acivicin	6	55
	13-cis RA	3	50
	DUP 937	0	50
	Elsamitrucin	0	72
	Tiazofurin	0	87
Glioma (first line)			
	Topotecan	8	**26***
	Docetaxel	0	**28***
	Gemcitabine	0	40
	Tiazofurin	0	69
	Trimetrexate	0	86

*Results which surpass the selection criteria noted in Table 4.

likely due to the ability of treatment to halt early PD not to cause regression. Other trials in the metastatic setting showed similar patterns in some, but not all tumor types.

These observations led to the question: can PD rate by itself be used in phase II studies to accept or reject interesting compounds appropriately? If so, this might be a useful tool for evaluation of those new drugs which are predicted to cause tumor stability. To pursue this we examined our phase II database to see if, using PD rate only, we would select the same agents for further study as identified by response rate. First we arbitrarily defined a maximum PD rate for the various tumor types assessed, above which the agent would be considered uninteresting (and therefore rejected from further study). Furthermore, the PD rate of interest might differ between tumor types. These steps are similar to the usual procedure for phase II stopping rules based on response when a minimum response rate is established to make an agent 'interesting' [9]. At present in designing phase II trials in untreated patient populations, higher response rates must be observed for a new drug to be selected in those diseases in which numerous agents are already available (e.g. breast or small-cell lung cancer) as compared to those tumor types with few effective treatments (e.g.: melanoma). The same logic ought to apply in assigning PD rates to select new agents. In table 4, minimum response rates have been assigned to breast, NSCLC and glioma tumors based on the general results of 'active' treatment and the usual phase II stopping rules. In addition, maximum PD rates have been assigned to the same tumors on the basis of what might be considered intuitively reasonable rates of progression that would make a new regimen more or less interesting. In table 5, results from a series of NCIC CTG phase II trials in each of these tumor types is shown in which the response and PD rate selection criteria have been applied. In all trials for each tumor type, the same patient eligibility and response criteria were used. As can be seen, regardless of whether response rate alone or PD rate alone would have been used, the same 3 agents would have been selected as 'interesting' in breast cancer. In NSCLC, the response rate criterion selected only 1 agent, while the PD criterion selected 2 (one of which was a paclitaxel combination regimen). Finally, in glioma although no agent met the response rate criterion, it is interesting to note that 2 agents (topotecan and docetaxel) have low PD rates.

These retrospective data suggest that the proportion of patients progressing early might be useful to select agents of interest for further evaluation. However, like all other alternative endpoints discussed, PD rate as a means of selecting new agents for phase III study remains non-validated. More work on all of these measures is needed to determine which, if any, are useful.

To return to the issue raised earlier: Is evidence of activity in phase II necessary before proceeding to phase III? Proceeding directly from phase I to phase III may to be a reasonable strategy in some circumstances, although it is risky. If pursued it would be most logical with agents where preclinical data is compelling and phase II results will not have an impact on plans to carry out randomized studies. The clinical settings in which such trials are done should be those where time to progression is relatively short and early stopping rules based on progression could interrupt the trial if appropriate. Examples might include the consolidation setting for treated small-cell lung cancer or ovarian cancer. Both of these are, in fact, being studied with metalloproteinase inhibitors.

Conclusions

In summary, this is time of tremendous opportunity in early clinical evaluation of anticancer therapy. Many potential new therapeutics have been designed to target the molecular mechanisms of cancer genesis, growth and metastases. Since some of these agents will be cytostatic rather than cytotoxic and since therapeutic doses may not need to be toxic, the traditional templates for phase I/II design and endpoints may not apply. On the other hand, adopting alternative endpoints simply because they are available is not to be advised if they are not validated in either mouse or man. Proposed new endpoints need prospective evaluation to determine their ability to correctly select drugs and doses that enhance survival, the final measure of true efficacy.

References

1 Rustin GJS, Nelstrop AE, Bolis G: Use of CA 125 to assess activity of topotecan versus paclitaxel in relapsed ovarian carcinoma measured by response and early progression. Proc Am Soc Clin Oncol 1997; 16: 351a(abstr).

2 Rasmussen H, Rugg T, Brown P: A 371 patient meta-analysis of studies of marimastat in patients with advanced cancer. Proc Am Soc Clin. Oncol 1997;16:429a(abstr).

3 Thalmann GN, Sikes RA, Chang SM, Johnston DA, von Eschenbach AC, Chung LW: Suramin-induced decrease in prostate specific antigen expression with no effect on tumor growth in the LNCaP model of human prostate cancer. J Natl Cancer Inst 1996;88:794–810.

4 Timothy AR, Cook GJR: PET scanning in clinical oncology. Ann Oncol 1998;9:353–355.

5 Zee B, Melnychuk D, Dancey J: A new design of phase II cancer clinical trials incorporating response and early progression. Controlled Clin Trials 1996;17:85S(abstr A80).

6 Dent S, Zee B, Dancey J: Design of phase II clinical trials – stopping rule using response and early progression. Ann Oncol 1996;7(S1):134(abstr).

7 Rapp E, Pater JL, Willan A, Cormier Y, Murray N, Evans WK, Hodson DI, Clark DA, Feld R, Arnold AM: Chemotherapy can prolong survival in patients with advanced non-small-cell lung cancer - report of a Canadian multicenter randomized trial. J Clin Oncol 1988;6:633–641.

8 Murray N, Coppin C, Coldman A, Pater J, Rapp E: Drug delivery analysis of the Canadian multicenter trial in non-small cell lung cancer. J Clin Oncol 1994;12:2333–2339.

9 Fleming TR: One sample multiple testing procedures for phase II trials. Biometrics 1982;38:143–151.

ONKOLOGIE

Onkologie 2000;23(suppl 3):7–8

Topotecan/Taxol in First-Line Small-Cell Lung Cancer: Where is the Benefit?

C.R. Tweedy Jr. D.F. Andrews III

Amos Cancer Center, Columbus, GA

Introduction

Small-cell lung cancer (SCLC) represents about 25% of all lung cancers in the United States at the time of diagnosis, with the number of new cases exceeding 40,000 in 1996 [1]. Unfortunately, due to its aggressive nature, between 60 and 70% of patients are found to have extensive stage disease (disease not fitting within one radiation field) at presentation. Most patients either present with or develop liver and brain metastases early in the course of their disease. In its untreated state, SCLC represents one of the most virulent cancers in medicine. Survival of SCLC at 5 years and thus apparent cure is rare (1–5%) [2, 3]. Standard therapies for patients with SCLC have been evolving over the past 3 decades. Initially patients were offered irradiation or surgery. Studies from the 1970s proved that combination chemotherapy prolonged survival 5-fold in comparison to surgery or irradiation alone. Essentially all patients with SCLC are offered some form of chemotherapy now. Irradiation continues to play a role particularly in patients with limited disease or for palliation in extensive disease (ED).

In ED SCLC, the standard chemotherapy has become the combination of cisplatin and etoposide because it offers an efficacy and toxicity benefit over cytoxan- and adriamycin-based regimens [4]. Several new agents have proven to be quite active, however, including ifosfamide (50% response), paclitaxel (34–41% response), gemcitabine (27% response), and topotecan (39% response). Combination regimens containing ifosfamide have been shown to have particularly good activity [5–7]. The study from the Hoosier Oncology Group [6] compared cisplatin, etoposide with and without ifosfamide and found 2-year survival rates favoring the addition of ifosfamide (13 vs. 5%).

As stated above, despite excellent response rates, long-term survivors are few in number. An analysis from the US National Cancer Institute recently showed no significant change in the duration of survival over the past 20 years in extensive SCLC [8]. This prompted the authors to conclude 'a reasonable approach would be to consider these patients for experimental therapy for initial induction with subsequent crossover to standard cisplatin-, etoposide- or cytoxan-based therapy if no response is achieved'. With this thought in mind, new agents and combinations have been studied.

Topotecan in SCLC

Topotecan is a semisynthetic analog of the alkaloid camptothecin and like camptothecin inhibits topoisomerase I. Topotecan is currently approved in the United States for second-line treatment of patients with SCLC and its approval is based in large part on the two studies described next. In the so-called 'Window of Opportunity' trial, topotecan was given intravenously (i.v.) over 30 min at 2.0 mg/m^2 in a daily ×5 schedule to treat chemotherapy-naive patients with advanced SCLC [9]. The response rate in the evaluable patients was 39% (7/18) with all responses being partial. This established early on that topotecan was one of the most active single agents for SCLC. A phase III study has demonstrated topotecan, given as a single agent at 1.5 mg/m^2 i.v. for 5 days, to be comparable to the 3-drug combination of cyclophosphamide/adriamycin/vincristine (CAV) in SCLC patients who had relapsed at least 60 days after completing first-line chemotherapy [10]. The overall response rate favored topotecan with 24 versus 18%. It was also shown that topotecan provided significantly greater symptom relief than CAV. There is currently a phase III trial (ECOG 7593) nearing completion of accrual using topotecan as a single agent (1.5 mg/m^2 i.v. for 5 days) in first-line therapy of extensive SCLC.

The Eastern Cooperative Oncology Group (ECOG) evaluated paclitaxel as a single agent in previously untreated patients with extensive SCLC [11]. Patients receiving paclitaxel 250 mg/m^2 i.v. over 24 h every 3 weeks. Of 32 evaluable patients, 11 (34%) had a partial response. Kirschling et al. [12] used the

KARGER

Fax +49 761 4 52 07 14
E-mail Information@Karger.de
www.karger.com

Accessible online at:
www.karger.com/journals/onk

Charles R. Tweedy Jr., MD
Ivinson Cancer Center
225 N. 30th Street
Laramie, WY 82072
Tel. +1 307 742-2141 or -2237, Fax -0334

same regimen combined with prophylactic G-CSF. Of 37 evaluable patients, 15 (41%) achieved a partial response. The activity of both topotecan and paclitaxel as single agents prompted a combination of these two agents.

In 1997, Jett et al. [13] reported the first data (phase II) of the combination of topotecan and paclitaxel in extensive disease SCLC. Topotecan was given at 1.0 mg/m^2 i.v. over 30 min daily × 5, followed by paclitaxel 135 mg/m^2 i.v. over 24 h on day 5 with G-CSF support. Cycles were repeated every 28 days. In 12 patients, a response rate of 92% was reported with 4 complete remissions. One-year survival was 50% and 2-year survival was 25%. This data was scheduled to be updated at the American Society of Clinical Oncology meeting in May of 1999. The Cancer and Leukemia Group B (CALGB 9430) has used the combination of topotecan 1.0 mg/m^2 i.v. for 5 days and paclitaxel 230 mg/m^2 i.v., day 1, in first-line therapy of extensive disease SCLC but observed 3 septic death and has subsequently lowered the taxol dose to 175 mg/m^2 with G-CSF support.

Starting in May 1997, our group at the Amos Cancer Center sought to confirm the Jett data with the exception that paclitaxel was given at 135 mg/m^2 i.v. over 3 h to conform to general community oncology practice [14]; all other doses and schedules were maintained. Growth factor support and prophylaxis with ciprofloxacin was used. Eligibility for entry was extensive disease, no prior therapy, performance status 0 or 1. A total of 15 patients have been treated with at least 6 cycles of chemotherapy and all are evaluable for response. Responses were assessed after every 2 cycles of chemotherapy. The overall response is 100% with 10/15 complete remissions and 5/15 partial remissions. In patients eligible for evaluation of 1-year survival, 8/10 are alive. The first patient treated in this study is alive and free of disease at 22 months. Responses have been rapid with almost all patients responding within 2 cycles. Toxicity was expected with grade 3 leukopenia occurring in 12/15, but no hospitalizations were required for neutropenic fever. No patients have discontinued therapy due to toxicity. Only 1 patient of the 15 has developed brain metastasis.

The combination of topotecan and paclitaxel is extremely active. It is too early in our study to assess the impact on 2-year survival but in this limited study population, it does have superior 1-year survival and overall response to previously studied regimens. The toxicity of this combination has also been easily managed. One has to be aware, however, that these were highly selected patients, all of whom had excellent performance status. A randomized trial of topotecan, paclitaxel versus cisplatin, etoposide is planned to assess the response rates and impact on long-term survival. It will also address the issue of whether topotecan may help to prevent brain metastases since topotecan does cross the blood-brain barrier and in our study did seem to be preventative or at least to delay onset of brain metastases.

Conclusions

SCLC continues to be a challenging malignancy, especially when the presentation is with extensive disease. The future improvements in survival are likely to come about with the delivery of new agents in unique combinations. Topotecan and paclitaxel, either in an alternating fashion or with other active agents or in combination with those agents, appear to be an important key to that improvement in survival.

References

1 Parker SL, Tong T, Bolden S, Wingo PA: Cancer statistics, 1996. CA Cancer J Clin 1996;46:5–27.

2 Johnson BE, Grayson J, Makuch RW, Linnoila RI, Anderson MJ, Cohen MH, Glatstein E, Minna JD, Ihde DC: Ten-year survival of patients with small-cell lung cancer treated with combination chemotherapy with or without irradiation. J Clin Oncol 1990;8:396–401.

3 Crown JP, Chahinian AP, Jaffrey IS, Glidewell OJ, Kaneko M, Holland JF: Predictors of 5-year survival and curability in small cell lung cancer. Cancer 1990;66:382–386.

4 Roth BJ, Johnson DH, Einhorn LH, Schacter LP, Cherng NC, Cohen HJ, Crawford J, Randolph JA, Goodlow JL, Broun GO, et al: Randomized study of cyclophosphamide, doxorubicin, and vincristine versus etoposide and cisplatin versus alternation of these two regimens in extensive small-cell lung cancer: A phase III trial of the Southeastern Cancer Study Group. J Clin Oncol 1992;10:282–291.

5 Loehrer PJ Sr, Rynard S, Ansari R, Songer J, Pennington K, Einhorn L: Etoposide, ifosfamide, and cisplatin in extensive small cell lung cancer. Cancer 1992;69:669–673.

6 Loehrer PJ Sr, Ansari R, Gonin R, Monaco F, Fisher W, Sandler A, Einhorn LH: Cisplatin plus etoposide with and without ifosfamide in extensive small-cell lung cancer: A Hoosier Oncology Group study. J Clin Oncol 1995;13:2594–2599.

7 Glisson B, Lee JS, Palmer J, Fossella F, Shin DM, Murphy WK, Perez-Soler R, Hong WK: Cisplatin, ifosfamide, and prolonged oral etoposide in the treatment of patients with extensive small cell lung carcinoma. Cancer 1998;82:301–308.

8 Chute JP, Venzon DJ, Hankins L, Okunieff P, Frame JN, Ihde DC, Johnson BE: Outcome of patients with small-cell lung cancer during 20 years of clinical research at the US National Cancer Institute. Mayo Clin Proc 1997;72:901–912.

9 Schiller JH, Kim K, Hutson P, DeVore R, Glick J, Stewart J, Johnson D: Phase II study of topotecan in patients with extensive-stage small-cell carcinoma of the lung: An Eastern Cooperative Oncology Group Trial. J Clin Oncol 1996;14:2345–2352.

10 Von Pawel J, et al: Topotecan versus CAV for the treatment of recurrent small-cell lung cancer: An Eastern Cooperative Oncology Group trial. J Clin Oncol 1999;17:658–667.

11 Ettinger DS, Finkelstein DM, Sarma RP, Johnson DH: Phase II study of paclitaxel in patients with extensive-disease small-cell lung cancer: An Eastern Cooperative Oncology Group study. J Clin Oncol 1995;13:1430–1435.

12 Kirschling RJ, et al: A phase II trial of paclitaxel and G-CSF in previously untreated patients with SCLC. Proc Am Soc Clin Oncol. 1994;13:326 (abstr).

13 Jett JR, et al: Topotecan and paclitaxel in extensive stage small cell lung cancer (ED-SCLC) patients without prior therapy. Lung Cancer 1997;18 (suppl 1):38(abstr).

14 Tweedy, Ball T, Andrews DF: Topotecan and paclitaxel in extensive stage small cell lung cancer as initial therapy. Proc Am Soc Clin Oncol 1999 (in press).

ONKOLOGIE

Onkologie 2000;23(suppl 3);9–12

Topotecan in Second-Line Therapy of SCLC: Impact on Survival?

R.M. Huber[1] U. Gatzemeier[2] H. Gosse[3] J. von Pawel[4] D. Hruska[5] J. Mezger[6] J.G. Saal[7] R. Kleinschmidt[8] C. Steppert[9] H. Steppling[10]

[1]Klinikum Innenstadt, Ludwig-Maximilians-Universität München, [2]Krankenhaus Großhansdorf, [3]Städtische Klinik Leipzig, [4]Zentralkrankenhaus Gauting, [5]Klinikum Schillerhöhe, Gerlingen, [6]St. Vincentius-Krankenhaus, Karlsruhe, [7]Malteser Krankenhaus. St. Franziskus-Hospital, Flensburg, [8]Medizinische Einrichtungen der Rhein. Friedrich-Wilhelms-Universität, Bonn, [9]Fachklinik Kutzenberg, Ebensfeld, [10]Clemenshospital, Münster for the SOABB Study Group

Introduction

Small-cell lung cancer (SCLC) accounts for about 25% of lung cancer at initial diagnosis. It is a highly chemosensitive disease, but despite high initial response rates, the median survival time is only 9–16 months in limited disease and 6–12 months in extensive disease [1, 2]. About 70% of the patients who have limited disease and over 90% of patients who have extensive disease will develop recurrent or progressive disease. There is no standard second-line therapy following first-line treatment, and the prognosis after relapse is poor [3]. CAV (cyclophosphamide, doxorubicine, vincristine) is often used after first-line treatment with etoposide and cisplatin. In two studies, CAV produced second-line response rates of 13 and 28% [4, 5], but duration of response to second-line chemotherapy is short, with a median survival time of 10–20 weeks [6].

Thus the identification of new, more active drugs is clearly crucial. Among several new drugs investigated during the last few years, topotecan has demonstrated significant activity. It is a semi-synthetic, water-soluble derivative of the alkaloid camptothecin, a specific inhibitor of the topoisomerase I. Inhibition of this enzyme results in cell-killing DNA damage during the course of DNA replication. It proves to be effective in patients with brain metastases and it may be effective in preventing brain metastases.

Topotecan passes the intact blood-brain barrier, and two phase II studies have already been performed in patients with relapsed or refractory SCLC with topotecan as a single agent at a dosage of 1.5 or 2 mg/m^2/day on 5 consecutive days [7, 8]. In a phase III comparison, the monotherapy with topotecan resulted in the same responses and survival as the combination of CAV, symptoms relief was significantly better with the topotecan treatment [9]. Additionally, Lane et al. [10] reported a significant longer survival for patients with stable disease after topotecan treatment compared to those with disease progression. Although in all studies topotecan therapy was well tolerated by the patients, the percentage of grade 3 and 4 hematological toxicities is high. Other clinical complications are rare, but dose reductions and treatment delays are required. In a study with a topotecan dosage of 1.25 mg/m^2/day published by Perez-Soler et al. [11], hematological toxicities such as granolocytopenia and thrombocytopenia grade 4 were observed in 28 and 11% of cycles, respectively.

As it became apparent by the analysis of Armstrong and O`Reilly [12] that the hematological toxicities are highest during the 1st cycle, the SOABB study group conducted a phase II study with an initial topotecan dose of 1.25 mg/m^2/day to reduce the hematological toxicities. In the following cycles the doses were increased or decreased depending on toxicities by a standard operational procedure.

Primary interest of this phase II study was median survival time of the patients, other objectives were the evaluation of the response rate and response duration of topotecan monotherapy in the second-line therapy of SCLC after platinum-based or non-platinum-based first-line therapy. The assessment of hematologic and non-hematologic toxicities and the assessment of the dose intensity were further objectives.

Patients and Methods

Eligibility Criteria

All patients were required to have a histologically or cytologically confirmed diagnosis of SCLC. They had to have first-line therapy and were categorized according to a platinum-based or non-platinum containing first-line therapy. At least one tumor lesion had to be measurable two-dimensionally. Other eligibility criteria included an Eastern Cooperative Oncology Group (ECOG) performance status of less than or equal to 2,

KARGER

Fax +49 761 4 52 07 14
E-mail Information@Karger.de
www.karger.com

Accessible online at:
www.karger.com/journals/onk

Prof. Dr. Rudolf M. Huber
Pneumologie, Medizinische Klinik
Ludwig-Maximilians-Universität München
Ziemssenstraße 1, D-80336 München (Germany)
Tel. +49 (0)89 5160-2590, Fax -4905
E-mail huber@medinn.med.uni-muenchen.de

corresponding to a Karnofsky index > 60%, a sufficient bone marrow and renal function and for women with childbearing potential an adequate contraception. All patients gave written informed consent before study entry.
Patients were ineligible if they had a history of first-line therapy with any topoisomerase I inhibitor, a history of other neoplasms than SCLC, surgery within the last two weeks prior to inclusion, or a history of hypersensitivity to topotecan. Also ineligible were pregnant or lactating women and patients with severe infections.

Pretreatment and Follow-up Studies

At the beginning and at the end of the study, all patients underwent a complete medical history. An assessment of performance status and staging were done at the beginning of the study, at the beginning of each cycle and at the end of the study. Blood counts were done at the beginning and at the end of the study, at the beginning of each cycle and during each cycle at day 8 and 15; blood chemistry was obtained at the beginning and the end of the study and at the beginning of each cycle.

Stratification

Patients were stratified in 2 groups based on first-line therapy, either failure after platinum-based chemotherapy or failure after non-platinum containing chemotherapy.
Retrospective strata include patients with sensitive or refractory disease as well as the duration of the remission of the first-line therapy.

Treatment Schedule

Topotecan was administered as a starting dose of 1.25 mg/m^2/day for 5 consecutive days every 21 days. Patients could receive a maximum of 6 cycles. Dose modifications were performed in steps by 0.25 mg/m^2/day based on hematological toxicity.
Grades of toxicity that occurred during the first treatment course will be reviewed and the dose for the next treatment course will be escalated by one step if only toxicities of NCIC CTCG grade 2 occurred.
The dose could be reduced in one of the following cases:

- NCIC CTCG grade 3 leukopenia (neutrophils 1.0×10^9/l) ≥ 7 days
- febrile neutropenia (T ≥ 38.2 °C and neutrophils < 0.5 and necessity of antibiotics)
- NCIC CTCG grade 3 thrombocytopenia (thrombocytes < 25×10^9/l)
- neutrophils < 1.5×10^9/l and thrombocytes < 100×10^9/l on day 22

The lowest dose level was 1.0 mg/m^2/day.
Re-escalation after dose reduction was not allowed.

Statistical Analysis

Data were analyzed by descriptive statistical methods.

Results

From March 1998 to January 1999 a total of 171 patients with recurrent SCLC were entered into the study from 43 German centers. The present evaluation is based on 100 patients, for whom complete data sets were available.
Main patient characteristics are listed in table 1. There were only 5% of the patients with limited disease, all other patients were extensive disease. Two thirds of the patients had a platinum-based first-line therapy, one third had mostly CAV or a modification of CAV as first-line therapy. Refractory patients was one third, and two thirds of the patients were considered sensitive with relapses between 3 and 6 months after first-line therapy. In first-line therapy patients had 23% complete remission (CR), 53% partial remission (PR), 5% stable disease (SD) and 19% progressive disease (PD).

Table 1. Main patient characteristics

	n	%
Eligible	171	
Evaluable	100	
Sex		
Male		75
Female		25
Age		
Median, years	60	
Range, years	38–76	
ECOG performance status		
0 (Karnofsky 100%)	16	16
1 (Karnofsky 80–90%)	59	59
2 Karnofsky 60–70%)	25	25
Extent of disease at study entry		
Limited disease	5	5
Extensive disease I	18	18
Extensive disease II	77	77
Brain metastases present	24	24
First-line therapy		
Platinum-based	66	66
Non-platinum-based	34	34
Time to relapse after first-line therapy		
< 3 months (refractory)	34	34
≥ 3 months to < 6 months (sensitive)	66	66
Best response to first-line therapy		
CR		23
PR		53
SD		5
PD		19

Dose Intensity

A total of 295 courses was given, the mean dosage was 1.28 mg/m^2/day. About 29% of the cycles could be increased to 1.5 mg/m^2/day, only 8.3% of the cycles had to be reduced to 1.0 mg/m^2/day. The mean dose density was (mg/m^2/day of a 21-day cycle) 0.26 in cycle 1, 0.3 in cycle 3, and 0.27 in cycle 5 (table 2).

Evaluation of Efficacy

The overall response rate was 14%. There were 14 patients (14%) with partial remission. 40 patients (40%) had stable

Table 2a. Mean dosage

	Total	Cycle					
		1	2	3	4	5	6
N	295	100	83	44	32	20	16
Mean dosage, mg/m²/day	1.28	1.25	1.29	1.33	1.39	1.38	1.39

Table 2b. Dose intensity

Dosage mg/m²/day	Patients		Cycles	
	n	%	n	%
1.0	13	13	24	8.3
1.25	59	59	180	62.5
1.5	28	28	84	29.2

Table 2c. Dose density

	Cycle				
	1	2	3	4	5
N	83	44	32	20	16
Dose density mean (mg/m²/day of a 21-day-cycle)	0.26	0.29	0.3	0.28	0.27

and 46 patients (46%) had progressive disease. We observed the same partial remission rate in platinum-based and non-platinum containing first-line therapy. There were little differences in the percentage of stable and progressive disease categories between platinum-based and non-platinum containing first-line therapy, this was also evident for performance status ECOG 0–1 and ECOG 2 (table 3). In 46% of the 24 patients with brain metastases, disease was arrested and 54% progressed.

The median time to progression for all patients was 8 weeks. Although there was a statistically significant difference regarding time to progression in those patients who could be increased with their dose (14 weeks time to progression), the median survival was equal. The 14 patients who responded had a median duration of response of 9 weeks.

The median survival time of all patients was 25 weeks. There were no differences between the type of first-line therapy or sensitive versus refractory. There was a difference in median survival time between the performance status: 25 weeks ECOG 0–1, 22 weeks ECOG 2.

Toxicity

The hematological side effects were remarkably rare with grade 4 neutropenia in 11.5% and thrombocytopenia grade 4 in 4.7% of the courses.

Table 3. Response rates

Response, %	All patients (n = 100)	Platinum (n = 66)	Non-platinum (n = 34)	ECOG 0–1 (n = 75)	ECOG 2 (n = 25)
CR	0.0	0.0	0.0	0.0	0.0
PR	14.0	14.0	15.0	12.0	20.0
SD	40.0	36.0	47.0	40.0	40.0
PD	46.0	50.0	38.0	48.0	40.0

Table 4. Comparison of time to progression and survival in relation to neutropenia and thrombocytopenia from the German multicenter study and the von Pawel study

	SOABB	Von Pawel et al. [9]	
Study drug	topotecan	topotecan	CAV
Median time to progression, weeks	8	13	12
Median survival, weeks	25	25	22
Neutropenia grade 4 (% of all courses)	11.5	38	52
Thrombocytopenia grade 4 (% of all courses)	4.7	10.3	1.5

At the dose levels of 1.25 mg/m²/day, there was grade 3 neutropenia in 12% and grade 4 neutropenia in 8%. Concerning the thrombocytes, there was grade 3 thrombopenia in 7% and grade 4 thrombopenia in 4%. The toxicities were not increased in those patients who could be increased during the course of their therapy, but they were lower in the dose levels of 1.0 mg/m²/day. There were no statistically significant differences concerning toxicities between the type of first-line therapy. Hematological toxicities were not cumulative during the course of the therapy.

There were few non-hematological side effects (fever: 2 patients, pancreatitis: 2 patients, dyspnoea, pneumonia, gastritis, erythema: 1 patient each).

Discussion

Prognosis in terms of response and survival of patients with recurrent SCLC still remains poor. Among several new drugs investigated during the last few years topotecan, a water-soluble analogue of camptothecin which acts as an inhibitor of topoisomerase I, has demonstrated significant activity. A phase II study conducted by the EORTC reported a 21.7% overall response (38% among sensitive, 6.4% among refractory patients) and a median duration of response of 33 weeks [7]. In that study the dose of topotecan was 1.5 mg/m²/day for 5 consecutive days, every 3 weeks. The remission rate observed in another study with topotecan as a single agent with 1.5 mg/m²/days 1–5 was 19% in sensitive patients and 3% in patients with refractory response to first-line therapy [8].

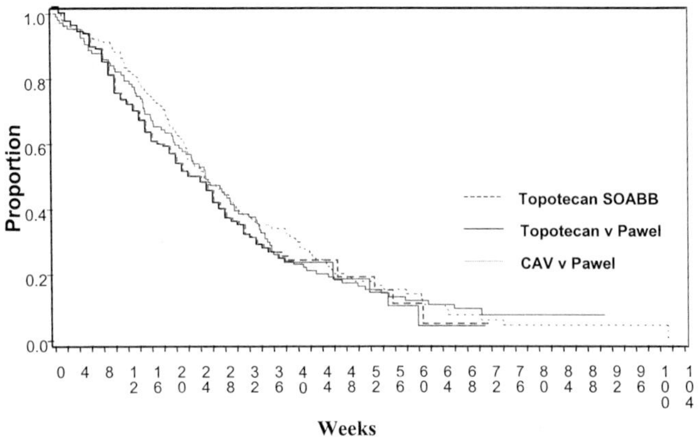

Fig. 1. Kaplan-Mayer plot for survival of both trials, German multicenter SOABB and von Pawel's study.

Perez-Soler et al. [11] already conducted a study with a topotecan dosage of 1.25 mg/m²/day. They recorded a remission rate of 11% (only partial remissions), 17% had stable disease and the median survival was 20 weeks.

Due to the promising results observed in these studies, a randomized phase III trial of topotecan as single agent versus CAV was performed [9]. In that multicenter trial, a total of 211 evaluable patients were included. As the patient characteristics are very similar to each other, a comparison of both studies is interesting (table 4). In the German multicenter trial the response rate achieved so far is 14% partial remission, the topotecan arm of von Pawel's study had 24%, the CAV arm 16%. The progression rate was 46% in the German multicenter trial versus 44.5 and 53% in the two arms of von Pawel's study. Although there were differences in the median time to progression (German multicenter study: 8 weeks, topotecan arm: 13 weeks, CAV arm: 12 weeks), the median survival time so far is 25 weeks for both topotecan arms, the dose adjustment for each patient in the German multicenter study and the standard dose of 1.5mg/m²/day in von Pawel's study, compared to 22 weeks in the CAV arm (fig. 1).

A comparison of the results regarding survival and myelotoxicity is summarized in table 4.

The topotecan dose modification could reduce myelotoxicity to half that of the standard treatment.

Thus in the German multicenter study presented here, there was the same efficacy and survival compared to a combination of 3 drugs with markedly less toxicity due to the lower starting dose of topotecan of 1.25 mg/m²/days 1–5 and subsequent dose modifications. Therefore topotecan has clearly an impact on survival in second-line therapy of small-cell lung cancer.

Appendix

The following institutions participated in this study:
Städtische Klinik Leipzig West, Krankenhaus Großhansdorf, Zentralkrankenhaus Gauting, Klinikum Schillerhöhe, Gerlingen, St. Vincentius-Krankenhaus, Karlsruhe, Malteser KRH St. Franziskus-Hospital, Flensburg, Clemenshospital, Münster, Fachklinik Kutzenberg, Ebensfeld, Med. Einrichtungen der Rhein. Friedrich-Wilhelms-Universität, Bonn, Krankenhaus Donaustauf, Klinikum Rechts der Isar, München, Medizinische Fakultät der Univ. Magdeburg, Diakoniekrankenhaus Halle, Klinikum der Albert Ludwigs-Universität, Freiburg, Krankenhaus Zschadraß, Zentral-Krankenhaus Bremen Ost, Zentralklinikum Augsburg, Mutterhaus der Borromäerinnen, Trier, Krankenhaus Nordwest, Frankfurt, Fachkrankenhaus Coswig, Klinikum der Hansestadt Stralsund GmbH, Allgem. Krankenhaus Hamburg-Harburg, Klinikum St. Marien Amberg, Universitätskliniken des Saarlandes, Homburg-Saar, Fachkrankenhaus für Lungen- und Thoraxchirurgie, Berlin, Krankenhaus Düren, Augusta-Krankenanstalt, Bochum, Kliniken Essen-Mitte , Klinikum Innenstadt, Ludwig-Maximilians-Universität, München, Klinikum Neubrandenburg, Klinikum Nürnberg, Krankenhaus der Barmherzigen Brüder, Regensburg, Städtisches Krankenhaus Bogenhausen, München, Städt. Krankenanstalten Krefeld, Klinikum der J. W. Goethe-Universität, Frankfurt, Universitätskrankenhaus Eppendorf, Hamburg, Städtisches Krankenhaus Heidehaus, Hannover, Städt. Klinikum Karlsruhe, Klinik Bad Trissel, Oberaudorf, Lungenfachklinik Philippstiftung e. V. , Immenhausen, Klinikum Chemnitz GmbH, Universitätsklinik, Jena, Universität Leipzig, Medizinische Universitätsklinik, Rostock

References

1 American Cancer Society: Cancer Facts & Figures. Atlanta, GA, American Cancer Society, 1997.
2 Minna JD: Neoplasms of the lung; in Isselbacher KJ, Braunwald E, Wilson, JD (eds): Harrison's Principles of Internal Medicine, New York, Mc Graw-Hill, 1994, pp 1221–1229.
3 Ihde DC, Pass HI, Glatstein EJ: Small-cell lung cancer; in DeVita VT, Hellmann S, Rosenberg SA (eds): Cancer, Principles and Practice of Oncology (ed 4). Philadelphia, PA, Lippincott-Raven, 1993, p 749.
4 Sculier JP, Klastersky J, Libert P: A phase II study evaluating CAVi (cyclophosphamide, adriamycine, vincristine) potentiated or not by amphotericin B entrapped into sonicated liposomes, as salvage therapy for small-cell lung cancer. Lung Cancer 1990;6:110–118.
5 Shepard FA, Evans WK, MacCormick R, Feld R, Yau JC: Cyclophosphamide, doxorubicin and vincristine in etoposide and cisplatin-resistant small-cell lung cancer. Cancer Treat Rep 1987;71:941–944.
6 Albain KS, Crowley JJ, Hutchins L, Gandara D, O'Bryan RM, Von Hoff DD, Griffin B, Livingston RB: Predictors of survival following relapse or progression of small small cell lung cancer. Cancer 1993;72:1184–1191.
7 Ardizzoni A, Hansen H, Dombernowsky P, Gamucci T, Kaplan S, Postmus P, Giaccone G, Schaefer B, Wanders J, Verweij J: Topotecan, a new active drug in the second-line treatment of small-cell lung cancer: A phase II study in patients with refractory and sensitive disease. J Clin Oncol 1997;15:2090–2096.
8 Eckardt J, Gralla R, Palmer MC: Topotecan (T) as second-line therapy in patients (pts) in small cell lung cancer (SCLC): A phase II study. Ann Oncol 1996;7:107(abstr 513).
9 Von Pawel J, Schiller JH, Shepherd FA, Fields SZ, Kleisbauer JP, Chrysson NG, Stewart DJ, Clark PI, Palmer MC, Depierre A, Carmichael J, Krebs JB, Ross G, Lane SR, Gralla R: Topotecan versus cyclophosphamide, doxorubicin, and vincristine for the treatment of recurrent small-cell lung cancer, J Clin Oncol 1999;17:658–667.
10 Lane SR, Fitts DA, Ross G, Fields SZ: Relationship between tumor response and survival in small-cell lung patients treated with intravenous topotecan as second-line therapy. Proc ASCO 1998;17:1896.
11 Perez-Soler R, Glisson BS, Lee JS, Fossella FV, Murphy WK, Shin DM, Hong WK: Treatment of patients with small-cell lung cancer refractory to etoposide and cisplatin with the topoisomerase I poison topotecan. J Clin Oncol 1996;14:2785–2790.
12 Armstrong D, O'Reilly S: Clinical guidelines for managing topotecan-related hematologic toxicity. Oncologist 1998;3:4–10.

ONKOLOGIE

Onkologie 2000;23(suppl 3):13–17

Topotecan in the First-Line Treatment of Small-Cell Lung Cancer

M. Wolf

Abteilung Innere Medizin, Institut für Hämatologie/Onkologie, Universitätsklinikum Marburg

Introduction

Little progress has been made in the treatment of small-cell lung cancer (SCLC) during the past two decades. While patients without metastasis currently have a 10–15% chance to achieve 5-year survival and the prognosis of this subgroup of patients has been improved in the last years by optimizing chemotherapy protocols and introducing multimodality treatment into therapy approaches, the prognosis of patients with distant metastases still remains very poor with a 3-year survival rate of less than 3% and nearly no chance of cure.

Furthermore, in extensive disease (ED) no improvement of treatment results has been observed in the last 25 years. Recently the Copenhagen Group [5] published an analysis of the prognosis of patients with ED treated between 1973 and 1981 compared to the prognosis of patients treated from 1982 to 1992. The median survival time of 508 patients included in the former studies was 208 days and not superior to the median survival of 215 days for 423 patients treated in the recent trials. Very similar results have been obtained in our study group. From 1981 to 1993 we performed 5 randomized trials including 738 patients with metastatic disease. The median survival time of the whole group was 234 days and the survival curves of these 5 consecutive trials were nearly identical and superimposable. The results of these trials led to the conclusion that the so-called standard chemotherapy regimens show a comparable activity in the subgroup of patients with metastatic SCLC and no particular drug combination seems to be superior to others. To overcome the present stagnation of treatment results in SCLC, the introduction of new drugs with a higher activity into treatment protocols is necessary.

In the last years several new drugs have been introduced to the treatment of metastatic SCLC. These comprise the taxans [6, 7], vinorelbine [8], gemcitabine [9], and the topoisomerase I inhibitors topotecan and irinotecan [10]. Among these new drugs, topotecan shows substantial activity in various malignancies such as ovarian cancer and lung cancer. This well-documented activity, even in tumors resistant to standard chemotherapy regimens [11], makes the drug especially interesting for testing in SCLC. This paper intends to summarize the currently available data about the activity of topotecan in first-line treatment of metastatic SCLC.

Single-Agent Activity of Topotecan in SCLC

There is currently one trial available, testing the activity of topotecan as single-agent first-line treatment in patients with ED SCLC. In this ECOG study from Schiller et al. [1] 48 patients with ED and without brain metastasis and prior chemotherapy were included and received a dose of 2 mg/m^2 as a 30-min infusion for 5 days. A total of 4 cycles were repeated in 3-week intervals. While the first 13 patients did not receive any hematopoietic growth factors, the other patients received G-CSF in a dose of 5 mg/kg body weight given from day 6 to 14 because of the substantial hematological toxicity seen in the first subgroup treated without growth factors.

In patients with progressive disease or in the case of no change after 2 cycles or partial remission after 4 cycles patients received further treatment with cisplatin 60 mg/m^2, day 1, and etoposide 120 mg/m^2, days 1–3, in 3-week intervals for further 6–8 cycles.

The hematological toxicity of the topotecan treatment is shown in table 1. Of the 13 patients treated without G-CSF, 77% suffered from a neutropenia WHO grade 4 and 38% from thrombocytopenia WHO grades 3/4. In the 35 patients treated subsequently with G-CSF, the hematological toxicity was markedly reduced and limited to a neutropenia WHO grade 4 in only 26%, while the incidence of thrombocytopenia WHO grades 3/4 was identical (37%).

Topotecan showed substantial activity in these patients with metastatic SCLC. 19 patients (40%) achieved a partial remission, no change was seen in 17 patients (35%), 6 patients showed progressive disease and 6 patients were not evaluable.

KARGER

Fax +49 761 4 52 07 14
E-mail Information@Karger.de
www.karger.com

Accessible online at:
www.karger.com/journals/onk

Dr. Martin Wolf
Department of Internal Medicine, Devision of Hematology/Oncology,
University Hospital
Baldingerstraße
D-35043 Marburg (Germany)

Table 1. First-line topotecan in ED SCLC [1]

Hematologic toxicity	Without G-CSF (n = 35), %	With G-CSF (n = 13), %
Neutropenia		
Grade 3	15	3
Grade 4	77	26
Thrombocytopenia		
Grade 3	15	20
Grade 4	23	17
Anemia		
Grade 3	15	23
Grade 4	0	9

Table 2. Treatment results of first-line topotecan in ED SCLC [1]

Best response	N	%
Complete remission	0	0
Partial remission	19	40
No change	17	35
Progressive disease	6	13
Not evaluable	6	13

The median progression survival was 3.9 months, the median survival time 10.0 months and the 1-year survival rate 39%. The results of the ECOG study are summarized in table 2.
These results outline the activity of the drug in the treatment of SCLC. The response rate is comparable to the activity observed in patients treated with paclitaxel and probably superior to the response rates seen after treatment with vinorelbine, irinotecan and docetaxel. These results of the single-agent activity provide the basis for the inclusion of topotecan into combination protocols for treating patients with metastatic SCLC.

First-Line Combination Chemotherapy in ED SCLC

The combination of topotecan with various additional cytostatic agents has been tested in a series of preclinical examinations in order to obtain information about synergistic or antagonistic effects. This preclinical data demonstrated a synergistic activity of topotecan in combination with alcylating agents [12]. Especially interesting in this setting were the combination of topotecan with cisplatin, which shows activity even in cisplatin-refractory tumors, and the combination of topotecan with etoposide. The target of etoposide is the enzyme topoisomerase II. In preclinical experiments, the activity of this drug combination depended strongly on the sequence of the drug administration. Concurrent application of etoposide and topotecan was connected with antagonistic effects while the sequential application – initial treatment with topotecan and subsequent etoposide application – resulted in synergistic activity. These results may reflect that topotecan pretreatment resulted in an up-regulation of the topoisomerase II levels which may be connected to higher sensitivity against the etoposide drug. This hypothesis has been clinically tested in patients with myelodysplasia and secondary leukemia [13]. In the treatment of these diseases, the topotecan-etoposide combination in the described sequential application showed an unexpected higher activity and has been identified as an active drug combination for treating these diseases.
Based on these preclinical investigations, first clinical experiences in SCLC have been made with the two drug combinations topotecan/etoposide and topotecan/cisplatin. Study designs and first results of these investigations will be described in the following section.

Topotecan/Etoposide in First-Line Therapy of ED SCLC

The Heidelberg Study

The sequential application of topotecan and etoposide has been tested in a dose-finding study performed by the Clinic of Thoracic Diseases in Heidelberg, Germany [2]. In this study, patients received topotecan in escalating doses starting with 0.5 mg/m^2 from days 1–5, followed by a fixed dose of etoposide of 75 mg/m^2 given on days 8–10. The dose of topotecan was increased in steps of 0.25 mg/m^2 per day up to a dose of 1.25 mg/m^2. Until now, 12 patients have been treated and the analysis of toxicity showed that the maximum tolerated dose (MTD) still has not been reached. In this setting, a dose level of 1 mg/m^2 for topotecan in the combination with 75 mg/m^2 etoposide was feasible without WHO grade 4 myelotoxicity. A definitive assessment of response and survival still has not been performed.

The Marburg Study

In the dose-finding study performed at our institution, we intended to shorten the whole treatment period in order to make the application of the chemotherapy protocol more convenient for the patients. Therefore, the topotecan application was restricted to 3 days and, after a 6-hour interval, followed by the application of etoposide in a dose of 80 mg/m^2 given from day 3 to 5. Topotecan starting dose level was 0.75 mg/m^2, days 1–3, and increased in increments of 0.25 mg/m^2 per day. The treatment plan in detail is shown in table 3.
Until now 7 patients have been treated using this protocol. The main characteristics of these patients are listed in table 4. All patients were males with metastatic disease. The

Karnofsky index was 70% in 3 cases, 80% in 3 cases and 90% in 1 case. Only 2 patients had a normal LDH level, in all other cases the LDH was elevated above the upper normal level of 240 U/l. Therefore, the whole patient population may be characterized by the presence of adverse prognostic features.

The performance of the treatment, the main hematological toxicity and the response of these patients are summarized in table 5.

Three patients received a starting dose level of 0.75 mg/m^2 topotecan for 3 days, 3 patients received the next dose level of 1.0 mg/m^2 and, until now, 1 patient received the 3rd dose level of 1.25 mg/m^2. In the starting dose level as well as in dose level 2, one patient each received only 1 cycle of treatment. In one case the further chemotherapy was refused, in the other case progressive disease was noticed after this first cycle. All the other patients received at least 4–6 cycles of the chemotherapy.

Until now, a WHO grade 4 myelotoxicity still has not been observed. In dose level 1, two patients experienced a WHO grade 3 leukocytopenia and 1 of these patients a WHO grade 3 thrombocytopenia. In dose level 2, none of the patients showed either a WHO grade 3 or 4 leukothrombocytopenia. During the course of treatment no cumulative hematological toxicity was observed. The clinical side effects of the treatment were very mild and none of the patients suffered from clinically apparent infections, peripheral neuropathy or moderate or severe nausea and vomiting.

Of the 7 patients, 1 had progressive disease after the 1st cycle resulting in premature stop of the treatment. In 3 further cases we observed a no-change and 3 patients achieved a partial remission of the disease. An analysis of survival is still to early and needs longer follow-up.

In conclusion the MTD of the 3 day topotecan application still has not been reached and further dose escalation will be performed.

Table 3. Study topotecan/etoposid (Marburg): Treatment schedule[1]

Dose level	Topotecan days 1–3, mg/m^2	Etoposide days 3–5, mg/m^2
1	0.75	80
2	1.0	80
3	1.25	80
4	1.5	80
5	1.75	80
6	2.0	80

[1]Six cycles in 3-week intervals.

Table 4. Study topotecan/etoposid (Marburg): Patients' characteristics

No.	Patient	Age, years	Sex	PS, %	Extent	LDH
1	K.K.	74	m	80	adrenal	278
2	K.K.	75	m	70	brain	223
3	K.B.	40	m	90	bone, liver, brain	368
4	G.M.	61	m	70	liver, abdominal, lymph node	465
5	H.M.	76	m	80	liver	468
6	E.H.	74	m	70	liver	310
7	A.S.	62	m	80	lung	230

PS = Performance status according to Karnofsky.

Table 5. Study topotecan/etoposid (Marburg): Results

No.	Dose mg/m^2	Cycles	Leukocytes nadir	Thrombocytes nadir	Anemia	Response
1	0.75	6	1.7	69	9.3	PR
2	0.75	1	4.0	170	12.4	NC
3	0.75	4	1.2	31	8.8	NC
4	1.0	1	4.4	210	11.7	PD
5	1.0	6	3.2	89	9.2	PR
6	1.0	4	3.3	110	11.3	PR
7	1.25	4	3.1	75	10.2	NC

PR = partial response, NC = no change, PD = progressive disease.

Combination Chemotherapy with Topotecan and Cisplatin

Cisplatin represents one the most active drugs for treatment of SCLC, and the combination of cisplatin with topotecan has shown synergistic activity in preclinical experiments. Therefore this drug combination may be especially interesting for treating this disease. However, first experiences in patients with non-small cell lung cancer (NSCLC) have shown a substantial myelotoxicity after application of topotecan over 5 days in combination with cisplatin on day 1. In the study of Wiesenfeld et al. [14], 83 patients with NSCLC were randomized to receive topotecan 1.25 mg/m^2, days 1–5, in combination with cisplatin 75 mg/m^2, day 1, or topotecan 1.0 mg/m^2, days 1–5, in combination with paclitaxel 190 mg/m^2, day 1. In this setting, 62% of the patients receiving the cisplatin-containing regimen experienced WHO grade 4 leukopenia and 76% WHO grade 4 thrombocytopenia. Therefore the patients recruitment in this treatment arm was stopped after 22 cases. An explanation for this unexpectedly high myelotoxicity of the combination topotecan/cisplatin was given by the work of Rowinski et al. [3]. These investigators treated 17 patients with different solid tumors with the combination of topotecan and cisplatin. These patients received topotecan in a dose of 0.75 mg/m^2 for 5 days and cisplatin in a dose of 75 mg/m^2 for 1 day. Cisplatin was given either on day 1 or 5 on alternate treatment cycles. The analysis of the hematological toxicity demonstrated that the application of cisplatin on day 1 was connected with a substantial increase of myelotoxicity in comparison to the cisplatin application on day 5. Further clinical trials of the combination topotecan/cisplatin took these results of Rowinski et al. [3] into account and tested the drug combination with cisplatin scheduled at the end of the topotecan administration.

The Copenhagen Trial

In the study of Sorensen et al. [4] from Copenhagen, the combination topotecan/cisplatin was used as a first-line treatment as part of an alternating treatment approach in patients with SCLC. 13 patients, 7 with limited stage and 6 with extensive stage, received topotecan in doses of 0.75–1.5 mg/m^2 for 5 days together with cisplatin 50 mg/m^2 on day 5 during the treatment cycles 1, 3, and 5. This regimen was alternated with a 4-drug protocol consisting of teniposide/carboplatin/vincristine/cisplatin given on cycles 2, 4, and 6. The dose of topotecan was escalated in steps of 0.25 mg/m^2 per day up to the highest dose level of 1.5 mg/m^2.

Up to now, 10 patients were evaluable for toxicity and response. In this trial, dose escalation up to the highest dose level of 1.5 mg/m^2 topotecan was feasible and did not result in an intolerable myelotoxicity. Of the 10 patients, 4 achieved a complete and 5 a partial remission resulting in an overall response rate of 90%. Therefore, in combination with cisplatin 50 mg/m^2 on day 5, the full dose application of topotecan was feasible.

The Marburg Trial

In the trial performed at our institution we restricted the topotecan application to 3 days and added the cisplatin on day 3. The main aim of the study was to determine the MTD of topotecan given for 3 days in combination with a fixed dose of cisplatin of 75 mg/m^2. Furthermore we intended to estimate the activity of this combination in the first-line treatment of SCLC.

The treatment schedule is given in detail in table 6. The starting dose level consisted of topotecan in a dose of 1.25 mg/m^2 for 3 days followed by cisplatin 60 mg/m^2 on day 3. Subsequently the dose of topotecan was escalated in steps of 0.25 mg/m^2 per day. In addition, the cisplatin dose was increased from 60 mg/m^2 (dose levels 1 and 2) to 75 mg/m^2 in dose levels 3–5.

Until now, 6 patients have been treated with this protocol. The main characteristics of these patients are summarized in table 7. All patients were male, 4 had a Karnofsky index of 80%, 2 of 90%. The median age was 58 years, all patients had metastatic disease and only 1 of the patients had a normal LDH level. Therefore the whole patient population can be characterized by the presence of poor prognostic features.

Of the 6 patients included, 1 received only 1 cycle of chemotherapy due to progressive disease. In the other patients, at least the dose escalation up to dose level 3, with 1.5 mg/m^2 topotecan for 3 days in combination with cisplatin 75 mg/m^2 on day 3, was feasible. The main hematological toxicity observed in these 6 patients is summarized in table 8.

From these preliminary results we conclude that the 3-day application of cisplatin in a dose of 1.5 mg/m^2 in combination with 75 mg/m^2 cisplatin given on day 3 is feasible. We are planning to increase the dose further in order to determine a MTD and to establish a 3-day regimen for cisplatin/topotecan in ED SCLC.

Table 6. Study topotecan/cisplatin (Marburg): Treatment schedule

Dose level	Topotecan days 1–3, mg/m^2	Cisplatin day 3, mg/m^2
1	1.25	60
2	1.5	60
3	1.5	75
4	1.75	75
5	2.0	75

Table 7. Study topotecan/cisplatin (Marburg): Patients' characteristics

No.	Patient	Age, years	Sex	PS, %	Extent	LDH
1	J.A..	68	m	90	bone, liver	327
2	H.F.	57	m	90	liver	231
3	R.P.	50	m	80	liver	2220
4	K.Z.	68	m	80	liver	329
5	A.H.	52	m	80	liver, lung	1670
6	K.H.	60	m	80	liver	420

Table 8. Study topotecan/cisplatin (Marburg): Results

No.	Cycles	MTD	Leukocytes nadir	Thrombocytes nadir	Anemia	Response
1	6	3	0.7	24	8.2	PR
2	6	n.r.	2.3	47	9.1	PR
3	1	n.r.	3.5	350	11.3	PD
4	3	n.r.	2.3	80	12.0	NC
5	3	n.r.	4.1	126	11.9	NC
6	2	n.r.	3.3	110	12.0	NC

PR = partial response, NC = no change, PD = progressive disease, n.r. = not reached.

Discussion

Topotecan is a new drug for treatment of SCLC which until now has been investigated mainly as a second-line treatment. In this setting, in phase II trials, the drug is able to achieve response rates up to 40% in sensitive tumors [15, 16]. This activity has been proven in the randomized trial from Pavel et al.

[17] comparing the topotecan second-line treatment to second-line standard CAV (cisplatin/adriamycin/vincristine) therapy. In this trial including 211 patients, the response rate for topotecan was 24% compared to only 17% for the CAV. Progression-free survival with 13.3 weeks vs. 12.1 weeks and overall survival with 24.7 weeks vs. 22.0 weeks were also slightly in favor for the topotecan treatment but did not reach statistical significance.

While the activity of topotecan in second-line treatment is well established, the currently available data about first-line therapy is still very limited. The only published first-line study with monotherapy of topotecan has been performed by the ECOG. In 48 patients a response rate of 40% was observed. This response rate is comparable to what was seen for second-line treatment of sensitive relapse. Furthermore this response rate is similar to the activity of other drugs which are widely used in treatment protocols for SCLC. Therefore topotecan represents one of the most active single-agent drugs for the treatment of this disease.

First experiences with combination treatments have been made together with etoposide, cisplatin, and paclitaxel. In combination with paclitaxel, Jett et al. [18] observed a very high response rate of 86% with a median survival time of 59 weeks and an 18-month survival rate of 26% in patients with metastatic disease. These data need to be confirmed by further investigations. For the combination treatment with etoposide or cisplatin, currently dose-finding studies are underway which concentrate on the establishment of tolerable and clinical feasible treatment schedules. In combination with a fixed dose of etoposide of 80 mg/m^2 for 3 days, a dose of topotecan in the range of 1.0 or 1.25 mg/m^2 for 5 or 3 days seems to be feasible. In combination with cisplatin, a sequence-dependent myelotoxicity is observed and the hematological side effects can be markedly reduced by application of cisplatin at the end of the treatment protocol. Using such a schedule, a dose of 1.25 mg/m^2 topotecan for 3 days combined with cisplatin 75 mg/m^2 given on day 3 seems to be feasible and clinical practicable. However, the activity of the combinations topotecan/etoposide and topotecan/cisplatin cannot be estimated in a reliable way until now. All these dose-escalating studies include only a small number of patients and focus on the evaluation of toxicity. Further patient enrollment in these dose-finding studies and subsequently the performance of phase II trials with fixed drug and dose combinations will be necessary in order to assess activity and survival of these drug combination of first-line treatment in SCLC.

References

1 Schiller JH, Kim KM, Hutson P: Phase II study of topotecan in patients with extensive-stage small cell lung carcinoma of the lung: An Eastern Cooperative Oncology Group Trial. J Clin Oncol 1996;14:2345–2352.

2 Buchholz E, Manegold C, Drings U, et al: Sequential administration of topotecan (TOPO) and etoposide (ETO) in extensive small cell lung cancer. Proc ASCO 1998;17:479a.

3 Rowinsky EK, Kaufmann SH, Baker SD, et al: Sequences of topotecan and cisplatin: Phase I, pharmacologic, and in vitro studies to examine sequence dependence. J Clin Oncol 1996;14:3074–3084.

4 Sorensen M, Jensen PB, Sehested M, et al: Phase I/II study of Topotecan and Cisplatin alternating with Carboplatin, Cisplatin, Teniposide and Vincristine in previously untreated patients with small cell lung cancer. Proc ASCO 1998;17:1931.

5 Lassen UN, Hirsch FR, Osterlind K, et al: Outcome of combination chemotherapy in extensive stage small cell lung cancer: Any treatment related progress? Lung Cancer 1997;18(suppl 1):6.

6 Ettinger DS, Finkelstein DM, Sarma RP, et al: Phase II study of paclitaxel in patients with extensive disease small cell lung cancer. J Clin Oncol 1995;13:1430–1435.

7 Burris HA, Crowley JJ, Williamson SK, et al: Docetaxel (Taxotere) in extensive stage small cell lung cancer (SCLC): A phase II trial of the Southwest Oncology Group (SWOG). Proc ASCO 1998;17:451a.

8 Depierre A, Le Chevalier T, Quoix E, et al: Phase II trial of navelbine (NVB), in small cell lung cancer (SCLC). Lung Cancer 1997;18(suppl 1):3.

9 Eisenhauer E, Cormier Y, Gregg R, et al: Gemcitabine is active in patients (pts) with previously untreated extensive small cell lung cancer (SCLC) – A phase II study of the National Cancer Institute of Canada Clinical Trials Group (NCIC CTG). Proc ASCO 1992;11:309.

10 DeVore RF, Blanke CD, Denham CA, et al: Phase II study of Irinotecan (CPT-11) in patients with previously treated Small Cell Lung Cancer (SCLC). Proc ASCO 1998;17:451a.

11 Creemers GJ, Bolis G, Gore M, et al: Topotecan, an active drug in the second-line treatment of epithelial ovarian cancer: Results of a large European phase II study. J Clin Oncol 1996;14:3056–3061.

12 Cheng MF, Chatterjee S, Berger NA: Schedule-dependent cytotoxicity of topotecan alone and in combination chemotherapy regimens. Oncol Res 1994;6:269–279.

13 Cooper BW, Lazarus HM, Creger R, et al: A phase I and pharmacodynamic study of sequential topotecan and etoposide (TE) in adult patients with refractory/Relapsed acute leukemia (RAL). Proc ASCO 1996;15:1549.

14 Wiesenfeld M, Marks R, Gril J, et al: A randomized phase II study of topotecan (TOPA) and cisplatin (CDDP) with filgrastim (G-CSF) versus topotecan and paclitaxel (Taxol®) with filgrastim in patients with advanced no-small cell lung cancer. Proc ASCO 1997;16:488a.

15 Ardizzoni A, Hansen H, Dombernowsky P, et al: Topotecan, a new active drug in the second-line treatment of small-cell lung cancer: A phase II study in patients with refractory and sensitive disease. J Clin Oncol 1997;15:2090–2096.

16 Perez-Soler R, Glisson BS, Lee JS, et al: Treatment of patients with small-cell lung cancer refractory to etoposide and cisplatin with the topoisomerase I poison topotecan. J Clin Oncol 1996;14:2785–2790.

17 Von Pawel J, Schiller JH, Shephard FA, et al: Topotecan vs cyclophosphamide, doxorubicin, and vincristine for the treatment of recurrent small-cell lung cancer. J Clin Oncol 1999;17:658–667.

18 Jett JR, Day R, Levitt M, et al: Topotecan and paclitaxel in extensive stage small cell lung cancer (ED-SCLC) patients without prior therapy. Lung Cancer 1997;18(suppl 1):13.

ONKOLOGIE

Onkologie 2000;23(suppl 3):18–20

Concluding Remarks

P. Drings

Thoraxklinik Heidelberg gGmbH

Small-Cell Lung Cancer

Small-cell lung cancer (SCLC) is characterized by a rapid tumor doubling time, a very high rate of cell proliferation as well as a tendency to early metastatic spreading. On the one hand, these biological properties are the reason for the poor prognosis of the tumor. On the other hand, they also account for a high sensitivity to chemotherapy and radiotherapy. With the introduction of chemotherapy, the median survival time of the patients was prolonged 5-fold and 5–10% of the patients survived for 3 years without recurrence. If one takes the group of patients with limited disease and other favorable prognostic factors, this percentage is indeed raised to 15–20%.

Whereas major advantages in treatment were not made during the last decade (or, putting it another way, consolidation was achieved at a very high level), it was nevertheless possible to obtain new insights into the importance of the various prognostic factors. On the basis of these factors, a distinction is made between a purely palliative therapy, e.g. in elderly patients with advanced tumors, and treatment with the primary objective of cure in patients with still limited tumor spreading.

Chemotherapy

Average rates of remission between 20 and 50% are attained with different cytostatics.

In the course of the 1970s, polychemotherapy became standard treatment, which is clearly superior to monotherapy because of high rates and longer durations of remission and longer survival times of the patients. As a rule, 2–4 cytostatics are administered simultaneously. In this way, it became possible to improve the patients' survival time substantially. In addition, the acute and chronic toxicity of the treatment could be greatly reduced by shortening the duration of treatment, by better selection of patients and consideration of newly defined prognostic factors as well as by replacing very toxic cytostatics with new substances. The combination of an anthracycline antibiotic (e.g. doxorubicin or epirubicin) with an oxazaphosphorine derivative (e.g. cyclophosphamide or ifosfamide) and a vinca alcaloid (e.g. vincristine) has been used for about 15 years. This widespread combination is known as the ACO or VAC schedule. In the meantime, there are several variations of this combination with regard to dosage and frequency of administration of the individual cytostatics. Alternatively, a combination of cisplatin or carboplatin with etoposide is used. When there is resistance to this treatment schedule or when individual cytostatics are contraindicated, several alternatives are available. Of these, in particular the combination cisplatin/etoposide has developed into the second standard procedure. However, the possible superiority of this combination compared to other schedules – especially when used in the stage of limited disease – that could be discerned in some studies could not be confirmed in the far advanced tumor stage of extensive disease.

Objectively measurable remissions are attained in 70 to more than 95% of cases with the combination of chemotherapy and radiotherapy in the stage of limited disease in patients who have not been pretreated. These include an average of 30–50% complete remissions. The actuarial survival times of all patients treated are specified as 12 months with certain variations between the individual studies. In complete remission, the actuarial survival increases to an average of 15–20 months. Whereas 40–70% of the patients have the chance of surviving for 1 year, only 10–20% of patients are free of recurrences after 2 years. This small percentage may be regarded as potentially cured.

In the stage of extensive disease, the rates of remission are very much less because of the substantially larger tumor mass. On average, the percentage of complete remissions does not exceed 20% and the median actuarial survival times of the patients are 6–9 months. One-year actuarial survival times of 20–50% are reported in the literature. Only very few patients survive without recurrences after 2 years.

KARGER

Fax +49 761 4 52 07 14
E-mail Information@Karger.de
www.karger.com

Accessible online at:
www.karger.com/journals/onk

Prof. Dr. P. Drings
Thoraxklinik Heidelberg gGmbH
Amalienstraße 5
D-69126 Heidelberg (Germany)

In past years, several attempts were made to intensify treatment. Examples of this are the administration of several agents, administration of consolidation or maintenance therapy, alternate administration of different combinations of cytostatics, continuos long-term treatment or high-dose therapy. Up to now, there have been no indications that simultaneous administration of 3 or 4 drugs is in principle superior to a dual combination. The duration of treatment has tended to be shortened to only 4–6 cycles, which could be discerned in recent years. Randomized therapy studies show that a short but very intensive chemotherapy engenders the same late results as a treatment of longer duration.

Maintenance chemotherapy subsequent to complete remission does not prolong the overall actuarial survival of patients. The same long-term result is attained with a 'wait-and-see' approach after complete remission and starting reinduction treatment if there is a recurrence. The appreciable efforts to validate the concept of alternate chemotherapy in SCLC made in the last decade did not reveal a convincing improvement of the results. The clinical experience that there are no major differences in efficacy between the established combinations in patients who have not been pretreated was confirmed. It is justified to continue treatment as long as the efficacy of every cycle can be proved.

An escalation of the dose in accordance with the concept of late intensification of chemotherapy in the form of consolidation treatment after complete remission has not yet shown any advantages. Extensive studies on the use of hematopoietic growth factors G-CSF and GM-CSF showed indications of better tolerance and lower toxicity of treatment. However, higher rates of remission and longer survival times could not be attained up to now. At present, investigations are being conducted as to whether the early positive interim results on high-dose therapy with stem cell substitution lead to a significant improvement of the late results.

Radiotherapy

Radiotherapy brings about a marked improvement in the results of therapy in SCLC. This is reflected in the 5-year actuarial survival times. A meta-analysis of Pignon et al. [1] comprising 2140 patients showed an improvement of the 3-year survival from 5.4 ± 1.4% for patients with irradiation of the thorax and a reduction of the annual risk of death by 14%. The value of radiotherapy in reducing local recurrences is manifested even more clearly. After chemotherapy alone, the rate of local recurrences is 60%. This value is halved by administering additional radiotherapy.

The probability of attaining local control by radiotherapy depends on the total dose administered and its fractionation. A total dose of at least 45–55 Gy is recommended.

In principle, chemotherapy can be administered before, after, alternately or simultaneously with radiotherapy in treatment of SCLC. One of the advantages in administering chemotherapy before irradiation is the diminution in size of the tumor, which permits a reduction of the irradiation volumes; in turn, this reduces the toxicity of the radiotherapy. As in administration after irradiation, the two treatment modalities can be administered at full dosage. Application of chemotherapy after irradiation might have the drawback that metastatic spreading outside the thorax might occur during radiotherapy which has a duration of roughly 5 weeks.

Simultaneous administration of chemotherapy and radiotherapy entails the risk of higher side effects and requires a fine adjustment of the doses of both treatment modalities. The toxicity of a combination containing anthracycline and/or cyclophosphamide is increased in a combined treatment schedule.

The therapy procedure with the greatest acceptance throughout the world consists in administration of polychemotherapy comprising 4–6 cycles, followed by consolidative irradiation of the thorax. Recent results of clinical studies indicate an improvement when the radiotherapy is administered earlier, i.e. simultaneously with the 2nd cycle of the chemotherapy. The reasons for the apparently better efficacy of early applied radiotherapy in the treatment of SCLC in the stage of limited disease are unclear at present.

Brain metastases are a special problem in SCLC. Patients surviving for a long time show a frequency of cerebral metastases of up to 80%. This is the basis for the idea of prophylactic radiotherapy of the brain, which has been the subject of controversy in the past. In several studies, a marked lowering of the rate of metastatic spreading into the cerebrum from 30–40% without prophylactic irradiation of the brain to 5–20% with prophylactic irradiation of the brain was demonstrated, although this did not lead to a prolongation of the patients' survival. However, a current meta-analysis of 987 patients by Auperin et al. [2] showed a significant improvement of the actuarial survival of patients with prophylactic irradiation of the brain. Three-year survival without prophylactic irradiation of the brain was 15.3% as compared to 20.7% with prophylactic irradiation of the brain. The most favorable time for this procedure has not been clarified.

Surgery

There has been a renaissance of surgery in SCLC in recent years after it had already be considered as obsolete by some oncologists. Surgery is justified as a supplementary measure to chemotherapy in stages I and II according tho UICC. However, less than 10% of all patients with this tumor meet this conditions. At present, the time sequence of surgery and chemotherapy in SCLC has not yet been unequivocally established even in the low tumor stages. Primary operation enables radical resection with immediate complete remission and thus good preconditions for adjuvant chemo/radiotherapy. On the other hand, the advantages of a secondary operation is that the active tumor tissue has been destroyed by the prior chemotherapy, the tumor is better encapsulated from the tumor-free tissue and possible distant metastases which could be demonstrated hitherto are eliminated.

References

1 Pignon JP, Arriagada R, Ihde DC, Johnson DH, Perry MC, Souhami RL, Brodin O, Joss RA, Kies MS, Lebeau B, et al: A meta-analysis of thoracic radiotherapy for small-cell lung cancer. N Engl J Med 1992;327:1618–1624.
2 Auperin A, Arriagada R, Pignon JP, Le Pechoux C, Gregor A, Stephens RJ, Kristjansen PE, Johnson BE, Ueoka H, Wagner H, Aisner J: Prophylactic cranial irradiation for patients with small-cell lung cancer in complete remission. Prophylactic Cranial Irradiation Overview Collaborative Group. N Engl J Med 1999;341:476–484.